Living with Lupus

Finding Strength and Resilience

Anna Brown

TABLE OF CONTENTS

CHAPTER ONE: INTRODUCTION

What is Lupus?

The autoimmune illness lupus is brought on when the body's immune system assaults its tissues and organs. Lupus-related inflammation can impact a variety of bodily functions, including your joints, skin, kidneys, blood cells, brain, heart, and lungs. Because of how frequently its signs and symptoms resemble those of other illnesses, lupus can be challenging to diagnose.

In many but not all instances of lupus, the most recognizable lupus symptom—a face rash that looks like butterfly wings expanding over both cheeks—occurs.

Some people are predisposed to lupus from birth, which can be brought on by illnesses, medications, or even sunshine. Lupus has no known cure, however, medicines can help manage symptoms.

Types of Lupus

Lupus comes in four distinct varieties. The kind of lupus that occurs most frequently is systemic lupus erythematosus (SLE). SLE is referred to as childhood-onset SLE, or cSLE if it manifests in childhood. 10 to 20 percent of SLE cases start while children are young. Most instances of SLE start between the ages of 15 and 44 as adults.

Cutaneous Lupus Erythematosus (CLE) is a less prevalent form of lupus that solely affects the skin. Acute Cutaneous Lupus, Chronic Cutaneous Lupus Erythematosus (Discoid Lupus), and Subacute Cutaneous Lupus are the three different kinds of CLE. The least frequent forms of lupus are drug-induced and neonatal.

Systemic Lupus Erythematosus

The kind of lupus that occurs most frequently is systemic lupus erythematosus (SLE). This is the kind of lupus that most people mean when they talk about lupus in general. Skin, joints, and kidneys are among the many organs that SLE can damage.

Cutaneous Lupus Erythematosus (Lupus of the Skin)
1. Acute cutaneous lupus
2. Chronic cutaneous lupus erythematosus, or discoid lupus erythematosus (DLE)
3. Subacute cutaneous lupus erythematosus

These types of Lupus is usually required to be diagnosed by a skin biopsy, because each has its own patterns and characteristic lesions.

<u>Chronic Cutaneous Lupus Erythematosus</u>

A rash that can leave significant scars is the primary symptom of chronic cutaneous lupus erythematosus, often known as DLE. Usually, it appears on your face, neck, and scalp. Less commonly, it appears on your upper chest and may also be on or in your ears. The margins of these scaly patches gradually grow larger before healing, leaving discolored skin and sunken scars. DLE on the scalp might result in long-term hair loss.

Drug-Induced Lupus Erythematosus

Taking specific prescription medications can result in this kind of lupus, which is distinct from SLE. Drug-induced lupus presents similarly to SLE, including joints and pulmonary inflammation.

Neonatal Lupus Erythematosus

Rarely, do newborns of mothers who have anti-Ro and anti-La antibodies get neonatal lupus. These maternal antibodies affect the infant's cardiac conduction system. The newborn may have a skin rash, liver issues, or a low blood cell count at delivery.

Symptoms and Diagnosis of Lupus

Symptoms

Lupus symptoms vary from person to person as well. For instance, a lupus patient can have a fever and swollen knees. Another person could experience chronic fatigue or renal issues.

Perhaps someone else has rashes. New symptoms may appear later on or some symptoms may become less frequent.

Additionally, lupus symptoms typically fluctuate, so you don't always experience them. The symptoms of lupus intensify during flares, which make you feel sick, and get better during remissions.

Lupus symptoms include:

Joint pain: Pain in the joints and muscles are lupus symptoms. You might feel stiffness and soreness together with or without swelling. Most lupus sufferers are impacted by this. The neck, legs, shoulders, and upper arms are typical locations for muscular soreness and edema.

Fever: Many lupus sufferers experience a temperature greater than 100 degrees Fahrenheit. Fever is frequently brought on by illness or inflammation. Fever can be managed and prevented with lupus medication.

Rashes: Any area of your body that is exposed to the sun, such as your face, arms, and hands, is susceptible to developing rashes. A crimson, butterfly-shaped rash that spans the nose and cheeks is one typical lupus symptom.

Chest ache: Lung lining irritation may result from lupus. When inhaling deeply, this results in chest discomfort.

Loss of hair: Bald or patchy areas are typical. Some medications or infections might also result in hair loss.

Sun or light sensitivity: The majority of lupus sufferers experience photosensitivity or sensitivity to light. Some lupus sufferers may get rashes, a fever, extreme exhaustion, or joint discomfort after being exposed to light.

Kidney issues: Lupus nephritis, which affects the kidneys, affects 50 percent of lupus sufferers. Weight gain, swelling ankles, elevated blood pressure, and impaired renal function are symptoms.

Mouth ulcers: These sores, also known as ulcers, typically develop on the mouth's roof but can also develop on the gums, inside the cheeks, and on the lips. You might have discomfort or dry mouth, or they could be painless.

Prolonged fatigue: Even when you get adequate sleep, you could still feel worn out or fatigued. Another indicator of an impending lupus flare is fatigue.

Anemia: Anaemia, a disorder that occurs when your body lacks red blood cells to transport oxygen throughout your body, might be the cause of your fatigue.

Memory issues: Some lupus sufferers claim to have memory loss or cognitive issues.

Clotting of blood: Your risk of blood clotting may be greater. Blood clots in the legs or lungs, a heart attack, a stroke, or recurrent miscarriages can all result from this.

Eye illness: You could get eyelid rashes, dry eyes, and eye irritation.

Diagnosis

Since there is no one test to diagnose lupus, your doctor will need to collect a lot of data using several methods, beginning with your medical history.

Your doctor will then do an examination and search for a few physical indicators of lupus. A biopsy, which is a technique to remove a little bit of your skin or kidney for microscopic inspection, may also be prescribed by your doctor. To determine whether and how your organs have been impacted, the doctor will also request blood, urine, and other tests.

Your doctor can use a variety of tests to assess whether you have lupus and, if so, how severe it is. Typically, you'll undergo the following exams. The information they obtain is all crucial information that can help with the diagnosis of lupus.

Lupus Diagnosis Tests

1. Complete Blood Count: A complete blood count (CBC) looks for low levels of platelets, white blood cells, and red blood cells.
2. Complement Deficiency tests: Tests measure complement levels in the blood, which are proteins

that aid in the eradication of foreign objects. Complement deficiency may be a sign of lupus.

3. Panel for chemistry: evaluates the health of your liver and kidneys.

4. The urine protein-to-creatinine ratio and urine analysis are used to check for renal lupus.

5. Tests for anti-dsDNA, anti-Sm, anti-RNP, anti-Ro, anti-La, antiphospholipid, and other autoantibodies associated with lupus.

CHAPTER TWO: THE EARLY DAYS OF LUPUS

The Emotional Toll of Lupus

Millions of individuals throughout the world suffer from the chronic autoimmune illness lupus. With lupus, the immune system assaults the body, including the brain and neurological system, rather than defending it. Mental and emotional health may be harmed by lupus and its therapies.

Living with lupus can cause emotional ups and downs. You could feel well one day and be bedridden with pain and exhaustion the next. Planning your life and explaining to others why you can't do the things you used to can be tough while dealing with the unpredictable nature of lupus.

The effects of lupus on the mind and body can be severe. Many lupus sufferers experience anxiety, sadness, and other mental health problems. It can be difficult to maintain optimism becauseof the ongoing pain and weariness, and the disease's unpredictability can be debilitating.

The effect lupus may have on your relationships is among the most difficult parts of the disease. Maintaining connections and communicating the situation to your loved ones can be tough when you have lupus, which adds to the disease's emotional toll. It's critical to understand the emotional toll that lupus takes and to get help when you need it.

For managing the emotional effects of the illness, consulting a therapist or joining a support group may be beneficial. It's crucial to have open lines of communication with your loved ones and to let them know what you need. Lupus can be difficult to live with, but it is possible to control its emotional effects.

Managing Stress with Lupus

Lupus may make daily life unpleasant. Additionally, stress might worsen or start your lupus symptoms. However, you may take action to reduce stress and safeguard your health.

Understand the symptoms and causes of your stress. Recognizing your symptoms is the first step in managing your stress. When under stress, you could experience:

1. Worry

2. Angry

3. Losing concentration

Physical signs like headaches or difficulties sleeping might also be present. Your lupus symptoms can also be becoming worse.

Next, consider the source of your stress. Do you experience tension, for instance, when you visit the doctor or while working? Consider maintaining a journal to record your stress-related symptoms and causes. You may then develop a strategy to manage your stress by being more conscious of what stresses you out.

Think ahead.

It may be calming and reassuring to plan for stressful circumstances and even routine jobs. Try the following tactics:

1. If your day is going to be hectic, make plans the night before for things like what to dress, what to eat for lunch, and how you're going to move about.

2. If you find going to the doctor stressful, prepare all of your questions in advance.

3. Try preparing what you'll say in advance if you're anxious about a business meeting or a challenging chat with a friend or loved one.

4. Additionally, if you have difficulties remembering your plans, jot them down in a notepad or the notes app on your phone so that you may relax and not worry about it.

Schedule some downtime.

When you're under pressure and pressed for time, unwinding might not seem important. However, getting some rest will help you have more energy for everything else on your list. Try the following advice:

1. Take time out to rest. Consider arranging a 20-minute break during the day or designating 1 day each weekend for pure relaxation.
2. Establish limits. Everyone needs a break from socializing, thus it's acceptable to decline invites.
3. Be sincere with your loved ones. The people who care about you will comprehend if you need to change plans or obligations to take care of your health.
4. When you set aside time to unwind, you could discover that doing nothing at all is the greatest course of action! Alternately, you may try soothing activities like:

a) Reading, viewing your preferred TV show, or playing some soothing music

b) Clearing your thoughts by doing yoga or meditation

c) Making art, writing, or engaging in another form of creativity

Create wholesome routines

Living a healthy lifestyle can help you manage your lupus symptoms and reduce stress. Develop these wholesome routines:

1. Get adequate rest. Sleep is essential for managing stress and your lupus symptoms.

2. Take action. You may immediately feel the benefits of physical activity in reducing stress!

3. Eat well. You can manage stress better when your body is receiving all the nutrition it needs.

Maintain your mental wellness.

Additionally, stress might increase your vulnerability to mental health issues including sadness and anxiety. And many lupus sufferers are impacted by these issues. According to research, persons with lupus frequently experience higher levels of anxiety and sadness than people without the disease.

Some remedies can assist, which is excellent news. Consult your doctor and develop a treatment plan if you suspect that you may be suffering from depression or anxiety.

Get assistance

You could feel overburdened and alone under stress. But keep in mind that you are not alone and that others can assist you. To get help, consider these suggestions:

1. Inquire with your medical team about stress management techniques, as well as about seeking mental health care or counseling.
2. Reach out to your loved ones; conversing with them and spending time with them will help you relax.

CHAPTER THREE: TREATMENT AND MEDICATION

Common Medications used to treat Lupus

Medicine is the major treatment for lupus. NSAIDs, corticosteroids, and other immune system-suppressing medications, as well as hydroxychloroquine and the most recent lupus medication, Benlysta, have all been tried to treat the disease.

Drugs for lupus function in various ways. The fact that they all lessen edema in the body is what they all have in common. Depending on your specific situation, you may require a single medication or a mix of medications.

NSAIDs. These typical medications, such as aspirin, ibuprofen, naproxen, or indomethacin, aid in reducing pain, edema, and stiffness. Some persons with relatively mild cases of lupus can manage symptoms on their own with NSAIDs.medications that fight malaria.

Researchers have discovered that the medication hydroxychloroquine (Plaquenil), which is used to treat malaria, also eases lupus flares. With mild to severe lupus patients, these medications are effective. They can aid in reducing lupus symptoms including skin rashes and joint swelling. But for severe lupus that affects the kidneys or other organs, hydroxychloroquine is not administered alone.

The adverse effects of the medications are often not severe, and they may help avoid problems, improving a person's long-term prognosis.

Benlysta. In 2011, Benlysta received approval to treat lupus in conjunction with existing lupus medications. Some lupus patients might lower their doses of steroids, which can have unsettling side effects, even if it does not assist all of them.

Benlysta, commonly known as belimumab, is an antibody that identifies and inhibits an immune system protein that aids in the body's cells being attacked by the immune system. The most frequent negative effects include diarrhea, fever, and nausea.

Corticosteroids. For lupus patients, oral steroids like prednisone and prednisolone can be a life-saving therapy. High doses of steroids can effectively manage symptoms during severe lupus flares that harm organs including the kidneys. But steroid side effects, such as depression, mood swings, and weight gain, can sometimes be bothersome or severe.

These medications have the potential to raise long-term risks for infections, weight-related illnesses including diabetes or high blood pressure, infections, and osteoporosis, and other bone issues.

Your rheumatologist will probably lower the dose as you improve. Some patients can quit taking steroids entirely, while others require long-term therapy with low-dose steroids.
Additionally, steroids are available as a topical medication that can be used to treat lupus-related skin rashes.

Immunosuppressants. Drugs that inhibit the immune system can help improve symptoms of lupus since the illness is brought on by an overactive immune system.

Azathioprine, cyclophosphamide, methotrexate, mycophenolate mofetil, and other strong medications are among them. They are often used when corticosteroids have failed or are not an option in patients with severe lupus. Because immunosuppressive medications prevent the body from fighting infection, they can have substantial adverse effects. When an infection or disease first appears, you should seek medical treatment if you use immunosuppressive medications.

Experimental and novel pharmaceuticals. Studies are being conducted on several lupus drugs, many of which are intended to target certain immune cells. Consult your doctor about participating in a clinical study if you're interested. different medicines.

Depending on their symptoms, many people with lupus require additional drugs because the disease may affect so many different body areas. Statins, diuretics, anticoagulants, bone-strengthening medications, blood pressure medications, antibiotics, stimulants, and other medications might be among them.

Remember that finding the ideal lupus medication or combination may take your rheumatologist some time. Additionally, if your symptoms alter over time, you could require various medications.

Alternative Therapies and Complementary medicine

A range of various medical and health care practices, systems, and goods known as complementary and alternative medicine (CAM) therapies are currently not regarded as a part of orthodox medicine. Alternative medicine is used instead of traditional treatment, whereas complementary medicine is used along with it. True alternative medicines are less often utilized, with most individuals using therapy as Complementary Medicines.

Vitamin A

A few examples of complementary and alternative medicine are Vitamin A, which is made up of retinol, retinoic acid, and beta-carotene. It is necessary for developing healthy gums, skin, and skeletons as well as for low-light and color vision.

Vitamin A deficiency is a widespread problem worldwide and the main factor in infantile blindness. It is simple to get vitamin A because it may be found in both plant and animal products, such as carrots, tomatoes, and broccoli.

There are few and few studies on vitamin A supplementation in human lupus. Patients with SLE may consume less vitamin A through their diets, but their blood levels do not. Vitamin A's ability to decrease pro-inflammatory cytokines while raising inhibitory ones has been linked to its ability to control immune system function

This is particularly clear in animal research on lupus, where vitamin A therapy prevents the development of the typical skin lesions associated with lupus. Skin lupus lesions disappeared after a week in one human trial of three lupus patients who received vitamin A.

Vitamin C

Supplementing with vitamin C may decrease the chance of developing cancer and shorten the length, but not the frequency, of the common cold. It is necessary for the manufacture of the stress hormone (catecholamine), as well as for cognitive processes like memory, and it can reduce oxidative stress.

The main justification for the use of vitamin C as a CAM appears to be this latter function. Through the process of "oxidative stress," which can lead to inflammatory tissue damage, the body's chemical reactions with oxygen create highly reactive free radicals that have a limited half-life.

Free radicals may harm lipids (often known as "fats"), including cholesterol, allowing oxidative damage and causing heart disease, or they may disrupt DNA, allowing the development of the well-known anti-DNA antibodies found in lupus.

According to research, SLE patients have decreased amounts of antioxidants that might prevent damage and inflammation, such as glutathione. Studies on SLE patients indicate that pro-oxidant processes are preferred over antioxidant ones because they correspond with disease activity.

Therefore, using antioxidants to balance this aspect of lupus makes some sense. Vitamin C (500 mg daily) and Vitamin E (800 IU daily) supplements for three months are correlated with lower levels of oxidative stress and lipid oxidation indicators, which may indicate a potential to lower cardiovascular risk or disease activity.

Vitamin D

A hormone called vitamin D is mostly produced by the action of sunshine on the skin. This is significant because people with lupus should stay out of direct sunshine. Vitamin D receptors are present in immune cells as well as the skin, kidney, and parathyroid glands, which suggests that vitamin D may have an impact on the immune system.

About vitamin D, there are two crucial questions. Can a low vitamin D level lead to autoimmune illness, first? According to extensive epidemiological research, those who consume more supplementary Vitamin D appear to have a decreased chance of developing multiple sclerosis and rheumatoid arthritis, which are both auto-immune diseases like lupus.

Vitamin E

Vitamin E is an antioxidant, just like vitamin C. Although there are various natural forms of vitamin E, only -tocopherol is required for human requirements. For both adult men and women, the recommended dietary intake is 22.4 units (15mg).

Mango, tomatoes, kiwi fruit, vegetable oils, nuts, seeds, and vegetable oils all contain vitamin E. Supplements with vitamin E frequently include more than 100 units, which is substantially more than the recommended daily allowance.

The quantity of crucial immune chemical messengers known as cytokines may be decreased by vitamin E. Additionally, it could lessen the oxidation of lipids like cholesterol, which might lessen the risk of cardiovascular disease.

Antioxidant vitamins may help prevent the illness or postpone its onset while lowering cardiovascular risk because inflammation is what causes extensive tissue damage in lupus and may raise cardiovascular risk.

In some immune cells employed to attack bacteria, lysosomes, which are containers containing corrosive enzymes, are stabilized with the aid of vitamin E. Because of their instability, lysosomes' enzymes can harm nearby healthy tissue. Therefore, vitamin E might delay the development of autoimmune damage.

N-acetyl Cysteine
N-acetyl Cysteine (NAC) is one of the other antioxidants. Medical applications for NAC include avoiding oxidative liver injury in paracetamol overdoses. It's a precursor of

glutathione, an antioxidant that occurs naturally but whose levels are low in the immune cells of SLE patients.

Omega-3 fatty acids

Omega-3 fatty acids and alpha-linolenic acid are found in flaxseed, which may assist to lessen inflammation. According to a preliminary study, flaxseed users with lupus may have healthier kidneys. This is crucial because a significant consequence of lupus is kidney disease, sometimes known as lupus nephritis. Before taking a flaxseed supplement if you also take blood-thinning medicine, such as warfarin (Coumadin), see your doctor.

Additionally, rich in omega-3 fatty acids, fish oil may aid lessen inflammation. The research on taking a fish oil supplement is conflicting.

However, medical professionals do advise lupus patients to consume more seafood. Fish from cold waters, such as salmon or halibut, are a good source. If you use blood thinners like warfarin (Coumadin) or other anticoagulants, consult your doctor before taking a fish oil supplement. Fish consumption does not carry the same danger.

Dehydroepiandrosterone

DHEA, or dehydroepiandrosterone. DHEA SHOULD NOT be taken without a doctor's approval. The body converts DHEA into the hormones testosterone and estrogen. Numerous clinical studies indicate that it could assist in reducing lupus symptoms. However, adverse effects were frequent and included acne, more facial hair, and excessive perspiration.

Additionally, DHEA may reduce HDL (good) cholesterol, which raises the risk of heart disease. People with a history of or increased risk of breast, uterine, ovarian, or prostate cancer should not use DHEA since it behaves like a hormone.

Methylsulfonylmethane

Methylsulfonylmethane (MSM) may aid in halting the deterioration of connective tissue and joints.

Importance of Working with a Healthcare Team

To effectively manage lupus, a healthcare team must be consulted. Rheumatologists, primary care doctors, nurse practitioners, and other experts may be on your team depending on your needs. They can provide you with the finest treatment, including prescription drugs, lifestyle advice, and emotional support.

To ensure that you receive the best care possible, it's critical to be upfront with your healthcare staff about your symptoms and concerns.

Some of the main advantages of collaborating with a medical team to treat lupus include the following:

Generalized care: Providing coordinated and integrated therapy that considers all facets of your health is how a healthcare team may provide comprehensive care. Together, they may create a tailored treatment strategy that takes into account your particular requirements and objectives. Medication, lifestyle advice, and emotional support are some examples of this.

A healthcare team can also assist you in managing the numerous lupus symptoms, including joint pain, exhaustion, and skin rashes. To assist you in overcoming the disease's emotional and social problems, they can also put you in touch with support groups and other services. A healthcare team's coordinated efforts can improve a patient's quality of life, reduce joint deterioration, and reduce flare-ups in lupus patients.

Personalized Care: By taking into consideration your particular requirements and goals, working with a healthcare team offers individualized care. You and your medical team can collaborate to create a treatment strategy that is customized for your unique circumstances. To make sure you get the best care possible, they might modify your treatment plan as necessary. Medication, lifestyle advice, and emotional support are some examples of this. You can get the individualized treatment you require to properly manage your lupus by working with your medical team.

Emotional assistance: To assist you in coping with the emotional and social issues of lupus, a medical team can connect you with services and support groups. They can also provide advice and therapy to assist you in controlling the stress and worry brought on by the sickness. Additionally, they can offer a secure and encouraging space where you can discuss your worries and emotions.

Access to new therapies: By keeping abreast of the most recent studies and clinical trials, a healthcare team can provide access to novel therapies. They can collaborate with you to decide if you qualify for novel therapies and guide you through the application procedure. To assist you in making an educated decision regarding your care, they can also give information about the advantages and disadvantages of novel therapies. You can get access to the newest, most potent lupus medications by working with a medical team.

Greater results: Working with a healthcare team can result in greater results since they can offer coordinated, integrated care that considers all facets of your health. Together, they may create a tailored treatment strategy that takes into account your particular requirements and objectives. You can get the individualized treatment you require to properly manage your lupus by working with your medical team. Better results, such as fewer flare-ups, less joint damage, and a higher quality of life, may result from this.

In conclusion, controlling lupus requires collaboration with a healthcare team. Your medical team can give you the best treatment available, including prescription drugs, lifestyle advice, and emotional support. Keep in mind that you are the most crucial member of your healthcare team, and the greatest results depend on your active engagement.

CHAPTER FOUR: NAVIGATING RELATIONSHIPS

Impact of Lupus on Family and Friends

The lives of family members and acquaintances may be significantly affected by lupus. It is a long-term autoimmune condition that can result in a variety of symptoms, such as joint discomfort, exhaustion, and skin rashes.

Families and friends may find it challenging to comprehend and assist their loved ones due to the unexpected nature of the condition. The impact on daily life is one of the most difficult parts of lupus for family and friends.

Lupus patients frequently feel weariness and joint discomfort, which can make it challenging to carry out daily duties. Family members who may need to take on more duties or offer care may feel the strain as a result. To meet the requirements of their loved one who has lupus, family members may also need to change their routines.

Family members and close acquaintances may also struggle with the emotional effects of lupus. Lupus patients may struggle with anxiety, despair, and other emotional issues.

Families may find it difficult to offer emotional support or may experience helplessness in the face of their loved one's difficulties. Stress, guilt, and frustration may result from this.

The unpredictable nature of lupus presents another difficulty for family and friends. Flares can happen at any moment, and their symptoms might change daily. Family members may find it challenging to schedule events or commit to responsibilities as a result.

It can also be challenging for friends to comprehend why a loved one might need to modify or cancel arrangements at the last minute. Despite the difficulties, there are several methods for friends and family to help a loved one who has lupus.

Learning more about the illness is among the most crucial things that family members can do. As a result, they will be more able to support their loved ones and comprehend the difficulties they are dealing with.

Family members can also help practically by doing housework or running errands for you. By hearing their loved one's worries and encouraging them, they may also offer emotional support. Similar assistance can be provided by friends, such as by running errands or just listening.

Additionally, friends and family must look after their own physical and mental well-being. It can be challenging to care for a loved one who has lupus, so it's critical to get help when you need it. This can entail going to therapy or joining a support group.

The lives of family members and acquaintances may be significantly affected by lupus. Daily living, emotional health, and relationships may all be affected. However, family and friends may assist a loved one who has lupus in managing the illness and leading a full life by providing them with information, practical assistance, and emotional support.

Family and friends may assist a loved one with lupus in overcoming the effects of the illness and achieving their objectives by working together. Encouraging the lupus patient to get medical attention and adhere to their treatment plan is one approach to offering assistance.

This can aid in symptom management and lower the likelihood of flare-ups. By supporting healthy behaviors like regular exercise and a balanced diet, family members may further assist. Additionally, it is crucial to have patience and understanding.

It might be challenging to anticipate how someone would be affected by lupus because it is a complicated disease. Flares can happen at any moment, and their symptoms might change daily. Family members should practice patience and understanding during this period. Supporting the lupus patient's ability to control their stress is another method to show your care.

Stress can cause flare-ups and exacerbate symptoms. By promoting relaxation practices like deep breathing or meditation, family members might be of assistance. They can assist by creating a serene and encouraging atmosphere.

Finally, it's critical to keep lines of communication open. Family members should urge their lupus-suffering loved ones to express their feelings. Additionally, they ought to be prepared to pay attention and offer help as required. Family members may make their loved one with lupus feel heard and supported by keeping lines of communication open.

Tips for Communicating with Loved Ones

Any strong connection starts with clear communication. It is a need if one of you has a chronic condition.

Play a proactive part

Communication is a two-way street, you've heard. With one speaking and the other listening, both parties are engaged. Make sure you are actively engaged, regardless of the part you are playing.

As you speak with your loved ones, take into account these suggestions:

Start your phrases with "I."

1. Ensure that you express your opinions and feelings clearly.
2. Never presume to understand another person's emotions.
3. Recognize that neither the other person nor anybody else can be changed.
4. Regardless of whether you can relate to or concur with the other person's sentiments, accept them.
5. Stay away from taking the victim's position.
6. A little humor can help, so use it.

7. Try to listen just as much as you speak, if not more.

8. Understanding your loved one should be your top priority.

Inform them of your lupus

It's crucial to be open and honest with the people you love about how you're feeling. Being open with your loved ones might allow them to better understand your situation and how they can support you.

The most important thing is to be open and honest with your loved ones, just like you would with your doctor. Yes, talking about your symptoms may get tiresome.

However, until you tell them, they won't be able to understand how you're feeling. There are some guidelines for discussing your lupus, whether you're in a new romantic relationship, with family members, or with an old acquaintance.

Define lupus.

Because lupus is a complex illness, it might be challenging for loved ones to comprehend what you're going through. Spend some time explaining to them what lupus is, how it affects you, and its symptoms. They may be more able to comprehend your demands and offer assistance as a result.

Describe your lupus management and treatment plan.
Tell them about the daily struggles you have and any lifestyle changes you've had to make as a result of your lupus. If it feels appropriate, go through your drug schedule.

Explain a lupus flare-up.
Living with lupus is unpredictable, which is one of the most difficult aspects. By explaining what a lupus flare is and how it affects you, you may prepare your loved one.

Discuss your triggers.
Verify that your loved one is aware of your triggers so they can assist you in avoiding them.
When you have lupus, it might be hard to communicate with your loved ones. Here are some pointers to assist:

Be persistent
Lupus symptoms might change from day to day and can be unpredictable. It's crucial to have patience with your family members and recognize that they might not always know how to assist. Give them time to pick up on your requirements and adjust.

Set limitations.

To keep your health in check, it's crucial to establish boundaries with your loved ones. Tell them if you need to take a break or if you don't feel like doing anything. Don't be scared to decline an offer if necessary.

Maintain contact

Because lupus may cause isolation, it's critical to maintain relationships with those you care about. Even if it's only a brief text or phone contact, try to remain in touch. Tell them how much you value their assistance.

CHAPTER FIVE: BALANCING WORK AND HEALTH

Challenges Working with Lupus

Working with lupus may be difficult since the disease's symptoms might be unexpected and necessitate frequent doctor visits or time off from work. Common symptoms that might make it challenging to concentrate on work or accomplish activities effectively include fatigue, joint discomfort, and brain fog.

Furthermore, stress can cause lupus flare-ups, so it's critical to control stress levels and engage in self-care. There are approaches to handling these difficulties, though. It's crucial to let your employer know about your health and any modifications you may want, such as a flexible schedule or remote work options.

Prioritizing rest and self-care is also crucial. You should also consult with your healthcare professional to manage your symptoms and stop flare-ups. Working with lupus and having a rewarding career are both feasible with the right management and assistance.

Working with lupus presents difficulties such as:

Managing unexpected symptoms
Working with lupus presents several difficulties, including managing unexpected symptoms. From moderate to severe, lupus symptoms might include weariness, joint discomfort, and mental fog. Both the employee and the employer may find it challenging to concentrate at work or accomplish duties quickly as a result of these symptoms.

Employees with lupus may need to modify their work schedules, take frequent breaks, or work from home to manage these symptoms. Employers must be patient, adaptable, and willing to collaborate with staff to discover solutions that benefit all parties.

Managing stress
Managing stress is a difficulty while dealing with lupus. Lupus flares, which can increase symptoms and need time off work to treat, can be brought on by stress. Employees with lupus must take measures to control stress, such as using relaxation techniques or scheduling frequent breaks during the workday. Employers may aid by fostering a positive work atmosphere and giving stress management tools like flexible scheduling or employee assistance

programs. Employers and workers can manage stress and avoid lupus flare-ups at work by cooperating.

Having conversations with employers

For workers with lupus, communicating with employers about the illness and any modifications that may be required can be difficult. Employers may be unaware of the illness or are unaware of the effects it might have on a worker's capacity for work. To develop solutions that work for everyone, employees with lupus may need to inform their employers about the illness.

A flexible work schedule, the option to work from home, or modifications to employment duties or obligations are all examples of accommodations. Employers may assist by being accommodating to employee requests and by educating managers and supervisors on how to support workers who have lupus at work.

Juggling work and rest

Striking a balance between work and rest is a struggle for people with lupus. Rest is crucial for treating symptoms, but it can mean missing work or rearranging your routine. To manage their symptoms, workers with lupus may need to take regular breaks throughout the day or work a modified schedule.

Employers may assist by creating a welcoming workplace that promotes flexibility and acknowledges the value of downtime. Employees with lupus can better control their symptoms and remain productive by taking regular breaks during the workday.

Organizing medical procedures and appointments

Lupus sufferers may have to coordinate their medication and treatment regimens while they are at work. This might involve controlling drug adverse effects, taking medications at specified times, or going to doctor's visits. Employers may assist by fostering a friendly workplace that allows for flexibility and acknowledges the need for medical care. To develop solutions that benefit everyone, employees with lupus may also need to discuss any restrictions or negative effects of their drugs with their employer.

Dealing with the disease's emotional effects

Setting self-care as a priority is one strategy for coping with the difficulties of living with lupus. This can involve getting adequate sleep, maintaining an active lifestyle, and eating well. Exercise can assist in managing lupus symptoms, but it's vital to see a doctor before beginning any exercise regimen. Employers may support employees by creating a supportive work environment that promotes self-care.

Examples of this include establishing wellness programs or flexible schedules that include work-related breaks for exercise or relaxation. Employees with lupus can manage their symptoms and continue to be productive at work by making self-care a priority.

Tips for finding a Work-Life Balance

Discuss Your Lupus with Your Employer: If you have lupus, it's crucial to discuss your illness with your employer and any adjustments you might require. This might involve having flexible work schedules, the option to work from home, or other perks that will make it easier for you to control your symptoms.

Manage Your Stress: Since stress can make lupus symptoms worse, it's critical to learn how to control your stress levels. This might involve engaging in relaxation practices like meditation or deep breathing, taking breaks throughout the day, and figuring out how to fit physical exercise into your daily schedule.

Establish a schedule: Establishing a schedule can assist you in controlling your lupus symptoms and preserving a positive work-life balance. This might involve designating time for work, other activities, and rest.

Reduce distractions and refrain from multitasking: It is simpler to focus when one subject at a time is the emphasis. Emails may be put on hold while you are working on a project. Alternatively, when you don't need to engage with clients or coworkers, use noise-canceling headphones.

Take it slow: When working on anything that takes focus, give yourself more time. Multi-step initiatives benefit from written project planning. If you require assistance, tell your manager or your coworkers.

Visual clues may be useful: Give yourself visible reminders if you frequently forget things. Put your headset next to your keyboard, for instance, to serve as a reminder to yourself that you have a recording to transcribe.

Prioritize: If you can, arrange your workday in advance. The most crucial activities should be highlighted so you may concentrate on them first. Plan your high-priority duties at times when you have the most energy if you tend to grow sleepy at particular times of the day.

Spend quality time in bed: You can start the day with as much energy as possible if you have a decent night's sleep. If you can, plan breaks throughout the day. Alter your surroundings or working hours. On days when you're feeling extra worn out, ask your manager if you may telework. If you often stand while working, try sitting for at least some of the time. If you are less energetic at some periods of the day, a flexible schedule could be helpful.

Hire assistance: Consider chores you can hand off so you may concentrate on important activities that demand your whole attention. Also, don't undervalue the importance of having a strong support system at home. This provides you additional leisure time so you may unwind and be well-rested for work.

Helpful machinery: A better chair might make a difference. Try voice-to-text technology if typing bothers your fingers. If you walk a lot at work, a mobility scooter could be an alternative.

Motion pauses. Pain can be lessened by even a little activity. Include many pauses for moving in the day. Avoid remaining still for extended periods of time.

Warm or cold treatments Heating pads provide pain relief for some people. Others discover relief from an ice pack. Consider keeping one of these accessible at work.

CHAPTER SIX: ADVOCACY AND AWARENESS

Ways to get involved in the Lupus community

To enhance access to care and therapies, boost public knowledge of the condition, and provide novel medicines, lupus advocacy and research are crucial.

Advocacy initiatives can aid in boosting research funding, enhancing patient care, and supporting laws that assist those with lupus, novel targets for therapy, a better knowledge of the disease's underlying causes, and the development of novel diagnostic tools can all be facilitated by research.

Participating in the lupus community if you or someone you know has the condition may be a terrific opportunity to meet new people, learn more about it, and improve the lives of those who have it. Here are a few ways to participate:

Join a group of supporters

Support groups can offer a secure and encouraging setting for people to interact with one another to share experiences, learn coping mechanisms, and live with lupus. Through the

Lupus Foundation of America or other lupus organizations, you can locate regional support groups.

Take part in lupus walks or other fundraising activities

To generate money for lupus research and activism, several lupus groups arrange fundraising activities including walks, runs, and bike rides. It may be enjoyable to take part in these activities and show your support for a worthwhile cause.

Volunteer

Volunteers are constantly needed by lupus groups to assist with fundraising, advocacy, and other tasks. Making a difference in the lives of those who have lupus and giving back to the community may both be accomplished via volunteering.

Advocate for lupus

By speaking with your political officials, posting about your experience on social media, and taking part in advocacy efforts, you can help spread the word about lupus and push for improved care and treatment.

Contribute to lupus charities

Contributions to lupus groups can be used to promote advocacy, support services, and research. Even tiny contributions can have a significant impact.

Self- and other-education

Increasing your knowledge of lupus can help you comprehend the condition and the effects it has on people's life. By enlightening people about lupus and its symptoms, you may further assist create awareness.

Participating in the lupus community can help improve the lives of those who have the disease and advance efforts to better understand and treat lupus in the future.

Raising Awareness about Lupus

The illness of lupus is complicated and frequently misunderstood. Even individuals who have heard of lupus may not completely comprehend what it is or how it affects people's lives.

An essential component of the battle against this chronic autoimmune illness is spreading knowledge about lupus. To spread awareness, try some of the following:

Tell your story

Nothing can be more credible than those who are advocating for a subject that they have personally experienced or have encountered via a loved one. To help others who may be experiencing these symptoms be identified sooner, share your story online, speak up in your community about your experience living with lupus, and educate people on the signs and symptoms of the disease.

Raising awareness and educating people about the disease can be accomplished by sharing your lupus story. You may tell your experience by speaking at events or support groups, posting it on social media, or publishing it in local newspapers or blogs.

Using Social media

Using social media to spread lupus awareness may be quite effective. To join the discussion and spread knowledge about the condition, use hashtags like #lupusawareness or #knowlupus. Additionally, you may disseminate articles, infographics, and other materials that inform others about lupus.

Host a gathering

Organizing an occasion like a walk, fundraiser, or educational session might be a terrific approach to increasing lupus awareness in your neighborhood. To assist in spreading the word and reaching a larger audience, you can work with neighborhood businesses or groups. Parties, garage sales, bake sales, and more may all be planned. These days, there are so many ways to raise money; all you need is the appropriate drive and a little imagination.

Put on purple

The hue of purple is used to symbolize lupus awareness. Purple attire and accessories can provide discussion starters and promote illness awareness. You may demonstrate your support by wearing purple ribbons or using other symbols.

One of the most popular items you can use to show your support and spread awareness about lupus is clothing and accessories. You may paint your toenails purple, wear a purple cap, or even construct your purple t-shirt—you get the point!

Inform others

The ideal advocate is knowledgeable. You may clarify misconceptions, respond to inquiries from the public, and further enlighten your friends, family, coworkers, etc. Many individuals may not be aware of what lupus is or have never heard of it. You may contribute to increasing awareness and promoting early diagnosis and treatment by teaching people about the illness and its symptoms.

Promote lupus funding and research

Promoting more funding for lupus research and care can aid in educating people about the condition and supporting initiatives to develop effective therapies and a cure.

CHAPTER SEVEN: LOOKING AHEAD

Advances in Lupus Research and Treatment

Because lupus affects immune systems differently in different people and has symptoms that can be mistaken for other illnesses, it is challenging to detect and treat. Additionally, the standard medications used to treat lupus have substantial adverse effects.

Doctors and researchers are nevertheless committed to identifying answers. The adverse effects of medications that have been standard therapy for decades are another distressing element of lupus. Prednisone is a common glucocorticoid used to treat the symptoms of lupus in individuals.

Although they have the potential to save lives, glucocorticoids can also have negative side effects including weight gain and osteoporosis. With the launch of the two new treatments that were authorized in 2021 and are especially aimed at lupus, doctors expect that situation will improve. These new treatments target particular molecules, unlike earlier therapies that were meant to inhibit the immune system overall.

Anifrolumab

In August 2021, Anifrolumab received approval. This monoclonal antibody is intended to treat an excess of interferon activation, which is crucial to the inflammation associated with lupus. A monoclonal antibody is a protein that searches for and binds to a particular kind of molecule, known as a cytokine, in the body. By intravenous infusion, it is given.

Voclosporin

Voclosporin, which received FDA approval in January 2021, is the first oral treatment for lupus nephritis. It functions by assisting in the inhibition of lupus nephritis-related inflammatory cell production while guarding against irreparable kidney damage.

Here are only a handful of the most recent therapy methods that are undergoing clinical trials:

B-Cell Treatments

The immune system in your body contains B cells. They serve as the body's army of tiny troops in the battle against pathogens. B cells release proteins called antibodies to combat foreign invaders like bacteria or viruses when they are detected. The B cells in your body turn against you when you have lupus. They produce antibodies that target the organs inside of you. Additionally, B cells produce substances that increase inflammation.

To treat lupus, a few new medications eliminate or stop B cells. Some of these medications are monoclonal antibodies, which are synthetic proteins that mimic the immune system's antibodies in function.

Monoclonal antibody obinutuzumab (Gazyva) kills B cells. Blood malignancies including follicular lymphoma and chronic lymphocytic leukemia (CLL) are already treated with it. Now, scientists are investigating if it may also cure lupus. The outcomes thus far are encouraging.

T-Cell Treatments

Another sort of immune cell that hunts for and eliminates pathogens is the T cell. Your T cells produce substances that worsen inflammation when you have lupus. Additionally, T cells instruct your B cells to produce more autoantibodies. Voclosporin (Lupkynis) was given FDA approval in 2021 to treat lupus nephritis. It prevents T cells from making the kidneys' immune system react. Tacrolimus (Prograf), which has previously received approval to reduce organ transplant rejection, disrupts T-cell activity. According to research, it may also be beneficial for lupus.

Plasma Cell Therapy

Autoantibodies are released by plasma cells, which are immune cells, in lupus. The existing lupus medications that suppress the immune system don't work effectively on these cells. Daratumumab (Darzalex), a cancer treatment, directly kills plasma cells. In one little research, daratumumab significantly reduced the severity of lupus symptoms. If this medication might be helpful in treating lupus, additional research is required.

Encouragement for those living with Lupus

Although managing lupus might be difficult, it's crucial to keep in mind that you're not alone. Many tools are available to help you manage your symptoms and enhance your quality of life if you have lupus, which affects millions of people worldwide. The most crucial thing you can do is to look after yourself. This includes getting enough sleep, eating well, and remaining active. Additionally, it's critical to control your stress levels because they might lead to flare-ups of lupus.

Think about engaging in relaxation methods like yoga, meditation, or deep breathing. Working closely with your medical team will help you manage your symptoms. Along with lifestyle modifications to make you feel better, your doctor could suggest medicines to help decrease pain and inflammation. Make sure to strictly adhere to your doctor's recommendations and advise them of any changes in your symptoms.

Keep in mind that lupus is a chronic disease that you will have to manage for the rest of your life. However, it is possible to live a full and meaningful life with lupus with the correct care and self-care. When you need help, don't be hesitant to ask for it, whether it comes from close friends and family, a support group, or a mental health professional. Finally, always remember to treat yourself well.

Even though dealing with lupus might be stressful and draining at times, it's crucial to keep in mind that you're trying your best. Don't be too harsh on yourself when things don't go as planned and remember to celebrate all of your accomplishments, no matter how minor. Finally, although managing lupus might be difficult, it's crucial to keep in mind that you're not alone. You can manage your symptoms and have a full and fulfilling life with lupus by taking care of yourself, collaborating closely with your medical team, and asking for help when you need it.